PLANT-POWERED POUNDS

Unlocking Weight Loss Success
through Vegetarianism

Dr. Raymond F. Bernard

TABLE OF CONTENTS

CHAPTER 1

Introduction to Vegetarianism and Weight Loss

In this opening chapter of our book, "Vegetarian Weight Loss Success," we dive into the fundamental concepts of vegetarianism and how it can be a powerful tool for weight loss. We'll explore the benefits, tackle misconceptions, and lay the foundation for your journey towards a healthier you.

Understanding Vegetarianism

First and foremost, let's clarify what being a vegetarian means. Simply put, a vegetarian is someone who doesn't consume meat, poultry, or seafood. However, vegetarianism isn't a one-size-fits-all lifestyle. It comes in various forms:

1. **Vegan:** Vegans avoid all animal products, including dairy, eggs, and even honey.
2. **Lacto-Vegetarian:** These individuals abstain from meat, poultry, seafood, and

eggs but consume dairy products.

3. **Ovo-Vegetarian:** Ovo-vegetarians avoid meat, poultry, seafood, and dairy but include eggs in their diet.

4. **Pescatarian:** Pescatarians primarily follow a vegetarian diet but include fish and seafood.

5. **Flexitarian:** This is a flexible approach where someone occasionally includes meat or animal products in their diet.

Now, you might wonder, why go vegetarian in the first place?

The Benefits of a Vegetarian Diet for Weight Loss

1. **Lower Calorie Intake:** Vegetarian diets tend to be naturally lower in calories than diets rich in meat and dairy. This can make it easier to create a calorie deficit, which is essential for weight loss.

2. **High Fiber Content:** Plant-based diets are typically high in fiber. Fiber not only keeps you feeling full but also aids in digestion and helps control blood

sugar levels, making it easier to manage your appetite.

3. **Rich in Nutrient-Dense Foods:** Vegetarian diets are often packed with nutrient-dense foods like fruits, vegetables, whole grains, nuts, and seeds. These foods provide essential vitamins, minerals, and antioxidants necessary for overall health.

4. **Lower Saturated Fat:** Vegetarians usually consume less saturated fat, which is commonly found in animal products. This can contribute to better heart

health and lower cholesterol levels.

5. **Improved Digestion:** Many plant-based foods are easier to digest than heavy, meat-centric meals. This can lead to better digestion and reduced bloating, which is beneficial for anyone looking to shed a few pounds.

6. **Ethical and Environmental Considerations:** Beyond personal health, adopting a vegetarian diet can align with ethical and environmental values. Reducing meat consumption

can help reduce the environmental impact of agriculture and animal farming.

Addressing Common Misconceptions

As with any lifestyle change, misconceptions and concerns can make the transition to vegetarianism seem daunting. Let's tackle some of the most common ones:

1. **Lack of Protein:** Many worry that vegetarian diets don't provide enough protein. While it's true that

meat is a concentrated source of protein, plants like beans, lentils, tofu, tempeh, and quinoa are excellent sources of plant-based protein. With proper planning, you can easily meet your protein needs as a vegetarian.

2. **Iron Deficiency:** Iron from plant-based sources (non-heme iron) is less readily absorbed by the body compared to heme iron found in meat. However, consuming iron-rich foods alongside vitamin C-rich foods can enhance iron

absorption. Leafy greens, lentils, and fortified cereals are good sources of iron.

3. **B12 Concerns:** Vitamin B12 is primarily found in animal products, so vegetarians, especially vegans, should consider B12 supplements or fortified foods. This is a manageable aspect of vegetarianism that ensures you get this vital nutrient.

4. **Taste and Variety:** Some worry that vegetarian meals will be bland or monotonous. In reality, a vegetarian diet opens the

door to a world of culinary possibilities. The variety of fruits, vegetables, grains, and legumes allows for endless creativity in the kitchen.

5. **Social Challenges:** Social situations, like family gatherings or eating out, can present challenges for vegetarians. However, with a bit of planning and communication, it's entirely possible to navigate these situations while sticking to your dietary choices.

Setting the Stage for Success

With these points in mind, it's essential to establish realistic expectations and set achievable goals for your vegetarian weight loss journey. Weight loss isn't about quick fixes or drastic measures; it's about making sustainable changes to your diet and lifestyle.

Understanding that there are various forms of vegetarianism allows you to choose a path that aligns with your preferences and values. Whether you go full vegan, embrace lacto-vegetarianism, or adopt a flexitarian approach, you have the flexibility to tailor your journey to your unique needs and circumstances.

Weight loss is not a one-size-fits-all endeavor, and it's crucial to remember that everyone's body responds differently to dietary changes. Therefore, while a vegetarian diet can be highly effective for weight loss, it's not a guaranteed magic solution. It's a tool—a powerful one—but how you use it matters.

In this book, we will guide you through every step of your vegetarian weight loss journey. We'll delve into meal planning, nutrient essentials, mindful eating, exercise, and overcoming common obstacles. By the time you finish this book, you'll be equipped with the knowledge and skills needed to embark on a successful vegetarian weight loss journey and maintain a healthier lifestyle for the long term.

So, let's start this exciting journey towards a healthier, more vibrant you. In the upcoming chapters, we'll dig deeper into the practical aspects of adopting a vegetarian diet for weight loss and provide you with the tools and strategies to achieve your goals. Remember, it's not just about losing weight; it's about improving your overall well-being and creating a sustainable, fulfilling lifestyle.

CHAPTER 2

Understanding Your Body and Weight Loss

In this pivotal chapter of our book, "Vegetarian Weight Loss Success," we're going to take a close look at the inner workings of your body and how weight loss fits into the equation. Understanding your body's metabolism, how it deals with calories, and the science behind weight gain and loss is fundamental to your success on this journey.

The Science of Weight Gain and Loss

Weight management boils down to a simple equation: the balance between calories consumed and calories burned. When you consume more calories than your body needs, the excess is stored as fat, leading to weight gain. Conversely, when you consume fewer calories than your body needs, it burns stored fat for energy, resulting in weight loss.

Your body's metabolism plays a crucial role in this process. Metabolism is the set of chemical reactions that occur within your cells to maintain life. It can be broken down into two primary components:

1. **Basal Metabolic Rate (BMR):** This is the energy your body requires at rest to perform essential functions like breathing, circulating blood, and maintaining cell function. It accounts for the majority of calories your body burns daily, around 60-75%.

2. **Physical Activity:** This includes everything from walking and exercising to simply fidgeting or tapping

your foot. Physical activity, or non-exercise activity thermogenesis (NEAT), can significantly impact your daily calorie expenditure.

Factors Influencing Metabolism

Several factors influence your metabolism, some of which you can control, and others you can't:

1. **Age:** Metabolism tends to slow down with age, primarily due to muscle loss. This makes it even more critical to maintain an active lifestyle as you get older.

2. **Gender:** Men typically have a higher BMR than women because they tend to have more muscle mass.

3. **Muscle Mass:** Muscle tissue burns more calories at rest than fat tissue, so the more muscle you have, the higher your BMR.

4. **Genetics:** Genetics play a role in determining your metabolic rate. Some people naturally have a faster metabolism than others.

5. **Hormones:** Hormones like thyroid hormones and insulin influence your metabolism. Hormonal

imbalances can impact weight management.

6. **Diet and Exercise:** Your food choices and activity level significantly affect your metabolism. Regular exercise can increase your BMR, and certain foods can boost metabolism temporarily.

Understanding these factors helps you appreciate that weight loss isn't solely about eating less; it's also about optimizing your metabolism through lifestyle choices and habits.

The Importance of Realistic Goals

Now, let's talk about setting realistic weight loss goals. It's essential to approach your weight loss journey with practical expectations to avoid disappointment and frustration.

1. **Sustainable Rate of Loss:** Aim for a gradual and sustainable weight loss of about 1-2 pounds per week. Rapid weight loss often involves drastic measures that are difficult to maintain long-term and can harm your health.

2. **Body Composition:** Shift your focus from just the number on the scale to your body composition. Building lean muscle while losing fat can result in a healthier and more toned physique, even if the scale doesn't change dramatically.

3. **Health Improvements:** Consider other health indicators beyond weight. Improved energy levels, better sleep, lower blood pressure, and reduced risk of chronic diseases are all valuable outcomes of a healthy lifestyle.

4. **Set Small Milestones:** Break your overall goal into smaller, achievable milestones. Celebrating these victories along the way can keep you motivated and on track.

5. **Non-Scale Victories:** Recognize and celebrate non-scale victories like fitting into old clothes, improved endurance, or increased flexibility. These can be just as rewarding as seeing a lower number on the scale.

Creating a Calorie Deficit

To lose weight, you need to create a calorie deficit, which means you're burning more calories than you consume. There are two primary ways to do this:

1. **Dietary Changes:** Reducing your calorie intake by making healthier food choices and controlling portion sizes.

2. **Physical Activity:** Increasing your level of physical activity to burn more calories.

Balancing Diet and Exercise

The most effective approach to weight loss combines both dietary changes and increased physical activity. Here's why:

1. **Diet:** Controlling your calorie intake through diet is critical because it's easier to reduce calorie consumption than to burn off excess calories through exercise alone. Plus, making healthy food choices provides essential nutrients for overall well-being.

2. **Exercise:** Incorporating physical activity helps you burn more calories, build

muscle, and boost your metabolism. It also offers numerous health benefits beyond weight loss, such as improved cardiovascular health, increased strength, and enhanced mood.

Mindful Eating and Portion Control

Mindful eating is an essential aspect of effective weight loss. It involves being present and fully engaged with your eating experience. By paying attention to your body's hunger and fullness cues, you can avoid overeating and make healthier choices.

Here are some tips for practicing mindful eating:

1. **Eat Slowly:** Chew your food thoroughly and savor each bite. Eating slowly allows your body to register when it's full, preventing overconsumption.

2. **Eliminate Distractions:** Turn off the TV, put away your phone, and focus solely on your meal. Distractions can lead to mindless eating.

3. **Listen to Your Body:** Pay attention to your body's hunger and fullness signals. Eat when you're hungry and

stop when you're satisfied, not when your plate is empty.

4. **Portion Control:** Use smaller plates and utensils to help control portion sizes. It's easier to avoid overeating when your plate isn't overflowing.

5. **Stay Hydrated:** Sometimes, thirst can be mistaken for hunger. Drink water throughout the day to ensure you're properly hydrated.

6. **Keep a Food Journal:** Tracking what you eat can help you become more aware

of your eating habits and identify areas for improvement.

The Psychological Aspect of Weight Loss

Weight loss isn't just about the physical aspects; it's also about the mental and emotional journey. Here are some psychological considerations:

1. **Motivation:** Identify your reasons for wanting to lose weight. Whether it's improved health, increased confidence, or a desire to be more active, having clear

motivations can keep you focused.

2. **Support System:** Share your goals with friends and family or consider joining a weight loss group. Having a support system can provide encouragement and accountability.

3. **Resilience:** Understand that setbacks and plateaus are a part of the journey. Developing resilience and the ability to bounce back from challenges is crucial for long-term success.

4. **Positive Self-Talk:** Replace negative self-talk

with positive affirmations. Be kind and patient with yourself throughout your journey.

In this chapter, we've explored the science behind weight gain and loss, the importance of setting realistic goals, and the need to create a calorie deficit through dietary changes and increased physical activity. We've also delved into the significance of mindful eating, portion control, and the psychological aspects of weight loss.

Armed with this understanding, you're better equipped to embark on your vegetarian weight loss journey. Remember, it's not just about losing weight; it's about embracing a healthier and more fulfilling lifestyle that supports your overall well-being. In the following chapters, we'll delve deeper into the practical aspects of adopting a vegetarian diet for weight loss, providing you with actionable strategies and guidance to achieve your goals.

CHAPTER 3

The Basics of a Vegetarian Diet

In Chapter 3 of our book, "Vegetarian Weight Loss Success," we're going to dive deep into the fundamentals of a vegetarian diet. We'll explore the various types of vegetarianism, provide guidelines for balanced vegetarian nutrition, and offer valuable tips for transitioning to this lifestyle. Understanding the basics of what you can and cannot eat as a vegetarian is a crucial step toward achieving your weight loss goals.

Types of Vegetarian Diets

One of the first things to understand about vegetarianism is that it's not a one-size-fits-all approach. There are several types of vegetarian diets, each with its own set of guidelines and food restrictions. Let's break down the most common types:

1. **Vegan:** Vegans follow the strictest form of vegetarianism. They exclude all animal products from their diet, including meat,

dairy, eggs, and even honey. A vegan diet is entirely plant-based.

2. **Lacto-Vegetarian:** Lacto-vegetarians avoid meat, poultry, seafood, and eggs but include dairy products like milk, cheese, and yogurt in their diet. This type of vegetarianism is prevalent in many cultures around the world.

3. **Ovo-Vegetarian:** Ovo-vegetarians abstain from meat, poultry, seafood, and dairy but include eggs in their diet. This provides an

additional source of protein and nutrients.

4. **Pescatarian:** Pescatarians are essentially vegetarians who include fish and seafood in their diet. They avoid other animal meats but consume fish for its health benefits, including omega-3 fatty acids.

5. **Flexitarian:** The flexitarian approach is the most flexible. Flexitarians primarily follow a vegetarian diet but occasionally include meat or animal products. This flexible approach allows

for a broader range of food choices.

Balanced Vegetarian Nutrition

Now that you know the various types of vegetarian diets, let's discuss how to maintain balanced nutrition while adhering to your chosen type.

1. **Protein:** Many people worry about getting enough protein on a vegetarian diet. However, plant-based sources of protein are abundant. Legumes like lentils, chickpeas, and black

beans, tofu, tempeh, seitan, quinoa, nuts, and seeds are all excellent sources of protein. Combining different protein sources throughout the day ensures you get a variety of amino acids, the building blocks of protein.

2. **Iron:** While meat is a good source of heme iron, which is readily absorbed by the body, vegetarians can obtain iron from plant-based sources. Leafy greens like spinach and kale, beans, lentils, fortified cereals, and tofu are rich in non-heme iron. To enhance iron

absorption, pair iron-rich foods with vitamin C sources like citrus fruits or bell peppers.

3. **Calcium:** Dairy products are a primary source of calcium for many, but lacto-vegetarians can get their calcium from milk, cheese, and yogurt. For vegans and those who don't consume dairy, fortified plant-based milk (e.g., almond milk, soy milk) and calcium-fortified foods are essential. Additionally, leafy greens like collard greens and bok

choy are naturally high in calcium.

4. **Vitamin B12:** Vitamin B12 is primarily found in animal products, so vegans should consider B12 supplements or fortified foods like plant-based milks and cereals. Lacto- and ovo-vegetarians can obtain B12 from dairy and eggs, respectively.

5. **Omega-3 Fatty Acids:** For pescatarians and those who include fish in their diet, omega-3 fatty acids are readily available. Vegans and other vegetarians can get their omega-3s from sources

like flaxseeds, chia seeds, walnuts, and algae-based supplements.

6. **Fiber:** Vegetarian diets are typically high in fiber, thanks to the abundance of fruits, vegetables, whole grains, and legumes. Fiber aids in digestion, helps control blood sugar levels, and keeps you feeling full, which can be beneficial for weight loss.

Transitioning to a Vegetarian Diet

If you're new to vegetarianism, transitioning to this lifestyle can be an exciting but sometimes challenging process. Here are some tips to make the transition smoother:

1. **Educate Yourself:** Learn about the different types of vegetarian diets and decide which one aligns best with your values and health goals.

2. **Gradual Transition:** You don't have to go vegetarian overnight. Consider gradually reducing your meat consumption while increasing your intake of plant-based foods.

3. **Explore New Foods:** Embrace the opportunity to try new fruits, vegetables, grains, and legumes. Experimenting with different recipes and cuisines can make the transition more enjoyable.

4. **Seek Support:** Connect with other vegetarians or join vegetarian groups and communities for advice, recipes, and support.

5. **Meal Planning:** Plan your meals to ensure you're getting a variety of nutrients. Include a mix of protein sources, whole grains, and

colorful vegetables in your diet.

6. **Read Labels:** Be vigilant about reading food labels, especially for hidden animal products and additives.

7. **Supplements:** If you're concerned about meeting all your nutrient needs, consider consulting a registered dietitian or nutritionist who can help you plan a well-balanced vegetarian diet and recommend appropriate supplements.

Why Choose Vegetarianism for Weight Loss

Now that you have a solid understanding of vegetarian diets and their nutritional aspects, you might wonder why choosing vegetarianism is a sound option for weight loss.

1. **Lower Calorie Density:** Vegetarian diets are often lower in calorie density, meaning you can eat more food for fewer calories. High-fiber, nutrient-dense foods like vegetables, legumes, and whole grains help you feel full and

satisfied while consuming fewer calories.

2. **Reduced Saturated Fat:** Many animal products, especially red and processed meats, are high in saturated fat, which can contribute to weight gain and heart disease. Vegetarian diets naturally contain less saturated fat, promoting heart health.

3. **Improved Insulin Sensitivity:** Plant-based diets have been associated with improved insulin sensitivity, which can aid in better blood sugar control

and reduced risk of type 2 diabetes—a significant factor in weight management.

4. **Enhanced Gut Health:** The high fiber content in vegetarian diets promotes a healthy gut microbiome, which can positively impact weight regulation and overall health.

5. **Long-Term Sustainability:** Unlike fad diets that are difficult to maintain, a well-planned vegetarian diet is a sustainable and enjoyable way of eating. This increases

the likelihood of maintaining weight loss in the long term.

In this chapter, we've delved into the basics of a vegetarian diet, including the different types, guidelines for balanced nutrition, and tips for transitioning to this lifestyle. Understanding what a vegetarian diet entails and how it can provide the nutrients your body needs is essential as you embark on your weight loss journey.

With this knowledge in hand, you're better equipped to make informed food choices, plan well-balanced meals, and enjoy the many health benefits that come with a vegetarian lifestyle. In the following chapters, we'll continue to explore practical strategies for achieving your weight loss goals as a vegetarian, helping you to create a sustainable and fulfilling path to a healthier you.

CHAPTER 4

Meal Planning and Preparation

Welcome to Chapter 4 of "Vegetarian Weight Loss Success." This chapter is all about the heart of your journey: meal planning and preparation. We'll delve into the art of creating balanced vegetarian meals, offer time-saving cooking tips, and provide you with sample meal plans and recipes to kick-start your weight loss adventure.

The Importance of Meal Planning

Meal planning is a cornerstone of successful weight loss. It's the proactive practice of deciding what you'll eat ahead of time, which not only saves you time and stress but also helps you make healthier choices.

1. **Controlled Portions:** Planning meals allows you to control portion sizes, reducing the likelihood of overeating. It also helps you avoid impulsive, less nutritious choices.

2. **Nutrient Balance:** Thoughtful meal planning ensures that you're getting a balanced mix of macronutrients (carbohydrates, protein, and fats) and essential micronutrients (vitamins and minerals).

3. **Reduced Food Waste:** By planning your meals, you buy only what you need, reducing food waste and saving money.

4. **Avoiding Decision Fatigue:** Making decisions about what to eat can be draining. Meal planning

eliminates the need to make those choices every day.

Building a Balanced Plate

A balanced vegetarian meal typically consists of:

1. **Protein Source:** Include plant-based protein sources like beans, lentils, tofu, tempeh, quinoa, nuts, and seeds. Protein keeps you full and supports muscle health.

2. **Complex Carbohydrates:** Opt for whole grains like brown rice, quinoa, whole wheat pasta, and oats. These provide sustained energy

and fiber, which aids digestion.

3. **Healthy Fats:** Incorporate sources of healthy fats like avocados, nuts, seeds, and olive oil. Fats contribute to satiety and support various bodily functions.

4. **Vibrant Vegetables:** Load your plate with colorful, non-starchy vegetables like leafy greens, peppers, broccoli, and carrots. These are rich in vitamins, minerals, and antioxidants.

5. **Flavorful Extras:** Use herbs, spices, and seasonings to enhance the

flavor of your dishes without relying on excessive salt, sugar, or unhealthy fats.

Time-Saving Cooking Tips

Cooking your meals at home gives you full control over ingredients and portion sizes. Here are some time-saving tips for efficient meal preparation:

1. **Batch Cooking:** Cook larger quantities of staple foods like grains, legumes, and roasted vegetables. Refrigerate or freeze portions for future use.

2. **Prep Ingredients:** Wash, chop, and prepare ingredients in advance, so they're ready to go when you're cooking.

3. **One-Pot Meals:** Prepare meals that can be made in a single pot or pan, minimizing cleanup time.

4. **Slow Cooker and Instant Pot:** These kitchen appliances are great for hands-off cooking. You can prepare stews, soups, and even whole grains with minimal effort.

5. **Sheet Pan Dinners:** Place a variety of vegetables and

protein sources on a sheet pan, drizzle with olive oil, and bake for an easy, flavorful meal.

6. **Mason Jar Salads:** Layer salads in mason jars with dressing at the bottom, followed by sturdy veggies and leafy greens on top. When you're ready to eat, shake the jar to mix the ingredients.

Sample Meal Plans and Recipes

Let's take a look at some sample meal plans to give you an idea of how to structure your meals:

Day 1:

- **Breakfast:** Overnight oats with almond milk, chia seeds, berries, and a sprinkle of nuts.
- **Lunch:** Chickpea salad with mixed greens, tomatoes, cucumbers, red onion, and a lemon vinaigrette.
- **Dinner:** Stir-fried tofu with broccoli, bell peppers, and a ginger-soy sauce, served over brown rice.

Day 2:

- **Breakfast:** Whole-grain toast topped with avocado,

cherry tomatoes, and a sprinkle of nutritional yeast.

- **Lunch:** Lentil soup with a side of whole-grain bread and a mixed greens salad.
- **Dinner:** Zucchini noodles with marinara sauce and homemade walnut pesto.

Day 3:

- **Breakfast:** Smoothie with spinach, banana, berries, plant-based protein powder, and almond milk.
- **Lunch:** Quinoa salad with black beans, corn, red onion, bell peppers, and a lime-cilantro dressing.

- **Dinner:** Baked sweet potato stuffed with black bean chili and a dollop of Greek yogurt.

These sample meal plans demonstrate the variety and deliciousness of vegetarian eating. Feel free to modify them based on your preferences and dietary requirements.

Experiment with Recipes

When it comes to recipes, the options are endless. Look for recipes that excite your taste buds and align with your nutritional goals. Explore vegetarian cookbooks, websites, and cooking apps for inspiration. You can find vegetarian versions of your favorite dishes, creative plant-based twists, and new flavor combinations to enjoy.

The Power of Preparation

In this chapter, we've explored the vital role of meal planning and preparation in your vegetarian weight loss journey. By planning your meals, you're setting yourself up for success—making mindful choices, ensuring balanced nutrition, and optimizing your time and resources.

Remember, the key to sustainable weight loss isn't just about what you eat, but also how you eat. Taking the time to plan and prepare your meals mindfully is a powerful step toward achieving your goals. In the upcoming chapters, we'll continue to provide you with the tools, strategies, and guidance you need to navigate your vegetarian weight loss journey with confidence and success.

CHAPTER 5

Nutrient Essentials for Vegetarian Weight Loss

In Chapter 5 of "Vegetarian Weight Loss Success," we're going to delve deep into the essential nutrients you need to pay attention to when following a vegetarian diet for weight loss. We'll discuss key nutrients that may require special consideration in a vegetarian lifestyle and provide guidance on how to ensure you get what you need through food choices and, when necessary, supplementation.

Protein: The Building Block of a Vegetarian Diet

Protein is a crucial nutrient for anyone, but it often takes center stage in discussions about vegetarian diets. It's the building block of cells, essential for muscle growth and repair, and it plays a significant role in weight loss.

Plant-based protein sources are diverse and nutritious:

1. **Legumes:** Beans, lentils, chickpeas, and peas are protein powerhouses.

They're versatile and can be used in a wide range of dishes.

2. **Tofu and Tempeh:** These soy-based products are rich in protein and can be marinated and cooked in various ways, making them a staple for many vegetarians.

3. **Nuts and Seeds:** Almonds, peanuts, chia seeds, and pumpkin seeds are not only protein sources but also provide healthy fats and fiber.

4. **Grains:** Whole grains like quinoa, bulgur, and farro contain some protein and

can complement other protein sources in your meals.

5. **Plant-Based Meat Substitutes:** Products like veggie burgers and meatless sausages can be convenient sources of protein, but it's essential to choose options with minimal processing and sodium.

Iron: Plant-Based Sources and Absorption

Iron is vital for transporting oxygen in the blood and maintaining overall health. There are two types of iron in foods:

heme iron (found in animal products) and non-heme iron (found in plant-based foods). Non-heme iron is less readily absorbed, but there are ways to enhance its absorption:

1. **Iron-Rich Plant Foods:** Leafy greens like spinach and Swiss chard, legumes, lentils, fortified cereals, and tofu are excellent sources of non-heme iron.

2. **Vitamin C:** Consuming foods rich in vitamin C (e.g., citrus fruits, strawberries, bell peppers) alongside iron-

rich foods can significantly boost iron absorption.

3. **Avoiding Inhibitors:** Certain compounds like tannins (found in tea and coffee) and calcium (found in dairy and fortified plant milks) can inhibit iron absorption. Try to consume these foods separately from iron-rich meals.

4. **Cooking in Cast Iron:** Cooking acidic foods like tomatoes or tomato sauce in cast iron cookware can increase iron content in your diet.

If you're concerned about iron intake, consider speaking with a healthcare professional or dietitian about supplementation.

Vitamin B12: Essential for Vegans

Vitamin B12 is vital for nerve function and red blood cell production. It's primarily found in animal products, so vegans need to be especially mindful of their B12 intake. Here's how to ensure you're getting enough:

1. **Supplements:** Most vegans will require a B12 supplement. These

supplements are widely available and safe. Speak with a healthcare provider to determine the right dosage for you.

2. **Fortified Foods:** Some plant-based foods are fortified with B12, including certain plant milks, breakfast cereals, and nutritional yeast. Check labels to identify fortified options.

Calcium: Beyond Dairy

Calcium is crucial for strong bones and teeth, and while dairy products are the primary source for many, vegetarians have several alternative options:

1. **Fortified Plant Milks:** Many plant-based milks (e.g., almond, soy, oat) are fortified with calcium and can be used in the same way as dairy milk.

2. **Leafy Greens:** Broccoli, bok choy, collard greens, and kale are excellent plant-based sources of calcium.

3. **Tofu:** Some tofu varieties are prepared with calcium sulfate, increasing their calcium content.

4. **Nuts and Seeds:** Almonds and chia seeds, for example, contain calcium and can be added to your meals or snacks.

5. **Fortified Foods:** Besides plant milks, other foods like fortified orange juice and breakfast cereals can contribute to your calcium intake.

Omega-3 Fatty Acids: Plant-Based Sources

Omega-3 fatty acids are essential for heart and brain health. While fatty fish like salmon are traditional sources of omega-3s, vegetarians can obtain them from plant-based sources:

1. **Flaxseeds:** Ground flaxseeds are an excellent source of alpha-linolenic acid (ALA), a type of omega-3 fatty acid. Sprinkle them on your cereal or blend them into smoothies.

2. **Chia Seeds:** These tiny seeds are rich in ALA and can be added to yogurt, oatmeal, or beverages.

3. **Walnuts:** Walnuts provide ALA and can be eaten as a snack or incorporated into

salads, oatmeal, or baked goods.

4. **Hemp Seeds:** These seeds contain a balanced ratio of omega-3 to omega-6 fatty acids and can be sprinkled on salads, yogurt, or incorporated into smoothies.

While these plant-based sources contain ALA, they may not offer the same benefits as the omega-3s found in fatty fish. Some vegetarians opt for algae-based omega-3 supplements to ensure they get the full range of these essential fatty acids.

Zinc: Plant Sources and Absorption

Zinc is crucial for immune function and wound healing. While animal products are rich in zinc, vegetarians can find it in plant-based sources:

1. **Legumes:** Lentils, chickpeas, and beans are excellent sources of zinc.

2. **Nuts and Seeds:** Pumpkin seeds, cashews, and almonds contain zinc.

3. **Whole Grains:** Oats, quinoa, and whole wheat products contribute to your zinc intake.

Like iron, zinc absorption can be influenced by phytates found in some plant foods. Soaking, sprouting, or fermenting these foods can enhance zinc absorption.

Iodine: Important for Thyroid Function

Iodine is essential for thyroid function and overall health. While iodized salt provides most people with enough iodine, some vegetarians may need to pay extra attention:

1. **Iodized Salt:** Use iodized salt in your cooking to

ensure you're getting enough iodine. However, be mindful of your salt intake, as excessive sodium consumption can be detrimental to health.

2. **Sea Vegetables:** Some sea vegetables like nori (used for sushi rolls) and dulse contain iodine. However, the iodine content can vary widely, so it's essential not to rely solely on sea vegetables for your iodine intake.

3. **Supplements:** If you're concerned about iodine intake, consider discussing

supplementation with a healthcare provider.

Supplementation: When and How

While it's ideal to get all your nutrients from food, some vegetarians may need supplements to ensure they meet their nutritional needs:

1. **Vitamin B12:** As mentioned earlier, most vegans should consider taking a B12 supplement.
2. **Omega-3 Fatty Acids:** If you're unable to get enough

omega-3s from food sources,
consider algae-based omega

CHAPTER 6

Vegetarian Weight Loss Strategies

Welcome to Chapter 6 of "Vegetarian Weight Loss Success." In this chapter, we'll explore practical strategies and tips to help you achieve your weight loss goals while following a vegetarian diet. Whether you're a long-time vegetarian or just starting this journey, these strategies will empower you to make informed choices, establish healthy habits, and stay motivated throughout your weight loss journey.

1. Portion Control and Mindful Eating

Portion control is a critical aspect of weight management. Here's how you can practice it:

- **Use Smaller Plates:** Choose smaller plates and bowls to help control portion sizes. A full small plate can feel just as satisfying as a half-empty large one.
- **Mindful Eating:** Pay close attention to your body's hunger and fullness cues.

Eat slowly, savor each bite, and stop when you feel comfortably satisfied, not overly full.

- **Avoid Distractions:** Turn off the TV, put away your phone, and focus solely on your meal. Distractions can lead to mindless eating and overconsumption.

2. Balanced Meals

Creating well-balanced meals is crucial for weight loss. A balanced meal typically consists of:

- **Protein:** Include a source of plant-based protein like

beans, lentils, tofu, or tempeh in each meal. Protein helps you feel full and supports muscle maintenance.

- **Complex Carbohydrates:** Opt for whole grains like brown rice, quinoa, and whole wheat pasta. These provide lasting energy and dietary fiber.

- **Healthy Fats:** Incorporate sources of healthy fats like avocados, nuts, seeds, and olive oil. Fats contribute to satiety and overall health.

- **Veggies:** Fill half your plate with non-starchy vegetables like leafy greens, broccoli, and bell peppers. These provide essential vitamins and minerals with fewer calories.

3. Plan Your Meals and Snacks

Meal planning and preparation are your allies in weight loss. Here's how to get started:

- **Weekly Planning:** Dedicate time each week to plan your meals and snacks. Create a menu and shopping list to ensure you have healthy options readily available.

- **Batch Cooking:** Cook large batches of staple foods like grains, legumes, and roasted vegetables. Refrigerate or freeze portions for future meals.

- **Healthy Snacks:** Have healthy snacks on hand, like cut-up veggies with hummus, fruit, or a small handful of nuts. Avoid keeping tempting, calorie-dense snacks in your home.

4. Monitor Your Intake

Keeping track of what you eat can help you stay accountable and identify areas for improvement. Consider these tracking methods:

- **Food Journal:** Write down everything you eat and drink throughout the day. Be honest and include portion sizes. Review your journal regularly to spot trends and adjust your habits.

- **Mobile Apps:** Use nutrition-tracking apps to record your meals and snacks. Many apps provide calorie and nutrient information, making it easier to stay on track.

- **Calorie Counting:** While not necessary for everyone, some individuals find calorie counting helpful for portion control. Remember that the quality of calories matters, so focus on nutrient-dense foods.

5. Hydration

Proper hydration is essential for overall health and can aid in weight loss. Here's how to ensure you're drinking enough water:

- **Water Before Meals:** Drink a glass of water before each meal to help control your appetite and avoid overeating.

- **Herbal Tea:** Enjoy herbal teas like green tea, peppermint, or chamomile. They can be a pleasant and hydrating alternative to sugary beverages.

- **Limit Sugary Drinks:** Avoid sugary sodas, energy drinks, and excessive fruit juices. These can add empty calories to your diet.

6. Regular Exercise

While diet plays a significant role in weight loss, regular physical activity is essential for overall health and can help you burn extra calories. Consider these exercise tips:

- **Find Activities You Enjoy:** Whether it's walking, jogging, cycling, dancing, or yoga, choose activities that you find enjoyable. You're more likely to stick with them.
- **Set Realistic Goals:** Start with achievable fitness goals and gradually increase the intensity and duration of

your workouts as your fitness level improves.

- **Strength Training:** Incorporate strength training exercises into your routine. Building muscle can boost your metabolism and help you maintain weight loss.

7. Stay Mindful of Healthy Snacking

Snacking can be a pitfall for weight loss, but it doesn't have to be. Here are some tips for healthy snacking:

- **Plan Snacks:** Include planned, nutrient-dense

snacks in your meal planning to prevent impulsive choices.

- **Portion Control:** Pre-portion snacks into small containers or bags to avoid overeating.

- **Choose Wisely:** Opt for snacks that combine protein and fiber, like yogurt with berries or whole-grain crackers with hummus.

- **Avoid Highly Processed Snacks:** Limit consumption of packaged snacks high in added sugars, salt, and unhealthy fats.

8. Mindset and Motivation

Your mindset plays a significant role in weight loss. Here's how to maintain a positive attitude and stay motivated:

- **Set Realistic Goals:** Establish achievable, specific, and time-bound goals. Celebrate your successes, no matter how small.

- **Practice Self-Compassion:** Be kind to yourself and recognize that setbacks are a natural part of the journey. Avoid self-criticism.

- **Visualize Success:** Imagine the positive changes in your life as you progress toward your weight loss goals.

- **Seek Support:** Share your journey with friends or join a weight loss group. Having a support system can provide encouragement and accountability.

9. Handle Social Situations Gracefully

Eating out or attending social events can pose challenges to your weight loss efforts. Here's how to navigate these situations:

- **Research Menus:** Before dining out, check the restaurant's menu online and choose a healthy option in advance.

- **Practice Portion Control:** Ask for a to-go box and portion out half of your meal before you start eating. This can help you avoid overeating.

- **Speak Up:** Don't be afraid to make special requests when ordering, such as dressing on the side or substituting fries for a side salad.

- **Stay Mindful:** Pay attention to your hunger and fullness cues, and stop eating when you're satisfied, even if there's food left on your plate.

10. Track Your Progress

Tracking your progress can help you stay motivated and make necessary adjustments to your plan. Here's how to monitor your weight loss journey:

- **Weighing:** Weigh yourself regularly, but don't obsess over daily fluctuations. Use your weight as one of many indicators of progress.

- **Measurements:** Take body measurements (e.g., waist, hips) in addition to weighing yourself. Sometimes, you may see changes in measurements even when the scale doesn't budge.

- **Non-Scale Victories:** Celebrate non-scale victories like increased energy, improved sleep, or fitting into old clothes.

11. Be Patient and Persistent

Remember that weight loss is not always linear. There will be ups and downs, but consistency and patience are key. Stay committed to your goals, and don't get discouraged by temporary setbacks.

12. Seek Professional Guidance

If you're struggling with weight loss or have specific dietary concerns, consider consulting a registered dietitian

CHAPTER 7

Overcoming Challenges in Vegetarian Weight Loss

In Chapter 7 of "Vegetarian Weight Loss Success," we address the common challenges you might encounter on your vegetarian weight loss journey and provide practical strategies to overcome them. Weight loss can be a rewarding but often challenging endeavor, and understanding how to navigate these obstacles can make all the difference in your success.

1. Plateaus and Slow Progress

Challenge: At some point, you may find that your weight loss progress has slowed down or even come to a halt. This is a common challenge in weight management.

Solution:

- **Reevaluate Your Caloric Intake:** As you lose weight, your body's caloric needs may change. Use a calorie calculator to determine if you need to adjust your daily intake.

- **Mix Up Your Workouts:** If you've been doing the

same exercise routine for a while, your body may have adapted to it. Try different forms of exercise or increase the intensity of your workouts.

- **Stay Patient:** Plateaus are a natural part of the weight loss process. Stay consistent with your healthy habits, and the scale will eventually reflect your efforts.

2. Emotional Eating

Challenge: Many people turn to food as a way to cope with stress, anxiety, or other emotions.

Solution:

- **Mindfulness Techniques:** Practice mindfulness techniques like deep breathing or meditation to become more aware of your emotional triggers for eating.

- **Emotional Journaling:** Keep a journal to track your emotions and food intake. This can help you identify patterns and make healthier choices.

- **Seek Support:** If emotional eating is a significant challenge, consider speaking with a therapist or counselor who can provide strategies for emotional regulation.

3. Social Pressures

Challenge: Social situations often involve food, and well-meaning friends and family may not understand or support your dietary choices.

Solution:

- **Communicate Your Goals:** Explain your weight loss goals and vegetarian lifestyle to your loved ones. Let them know how they can support you, such as choosing restaurants with vegetarian options when dining out.

- **Be Prepared:** Bring your own vegetarian dishes to social gatherings or eat a small, healthy meal before attending, so you're less tempted by unhealthy options.

- **Lead by Example:** Show your friends and family that a vegetarian diet can be delicious and satisfying by preparing and sharing tasty vegetarian meals with them.

4. Dining Out

Challenge: Dining out can be a challenge when trying to stick to a healthy, vegetarian diet.

Solution:

- **Research Restaurants:** Before going out, research restaurants in your area that offer vegetarian or vegan options. Many restaurants now have dedicated vegetarian menus.

- **Modify Menu Items:** Don't be afraid to ask for modifications to dishes. For example, you can request a salad without cheese or dressing on the side.

- **Portion Control:** Restaurant portions are often larger than what you need. Consider sharing dishes or boxing up half your meal to take home.

5. Cravings and Temptations

Challenge: Cravings for unhealthy foods can be a significant obstacle to weight loss.

Solution:

- **Healthy Substitutes:** Find healthier alternatives to your favorite indulgent foods. For example, if you're craving something sweet, opt for a piece of fruit or a small serving of dark chocolate.

- **Practice Moderation:** It's okay to indulge occasionally, but practice moderation. Enjoy a small portion of your favorite treat rather than overindulging.

- **Stay Hydrated:** Sometimes, thirst can be mistaken for hunger. Drink water when you have a craving and see if it subsides.

6. Nutritional Gaps

Challenge: Ensuring you get all the essential nutrients on a vegetarian diet can be challenging, especially for new vegetarians.

Solution:

- **Consult a Dietitian:** A registered dietitian can help you create a balanced meal plan that meets your nutritional needs.

- **Supplements:** If you're concerned about nutrient gaps, consider supplements like B12, vitamin D, or omega-3 fatty acids, but only after consulting a healthcare professional.

- **Variety Is Key:** Ensure you're eating a wide variety of fruits, vegetables, grains, legumes, nuts, and seeds to cover your nutritional bases.

7. Time Constraints

Challenge: Busy schedules can make it challenging to prioritize healthy eating and regular exercise.

Solution:

- **Meal Prep:** Dedicate some time each week to meal prep. Cook in batches and freeze portions for busy days.

- **Short Workouts:** You don't need hours at the gym. Short, high-intensity workouts or even 30-minute daily walks can be effective for weight loss.

- **Prioritize Self-Care:** Make self-care a priority, as stress can hinder weight loss progress. Set aside time for relaxation and stress management.

8. Weight Loss Plateaus

Challenge: At some point, you may hit a plateau where your weight loss stalls despite your efforts.

Solution:

- **Review Your Habits:** Reevaluate your dietary and exercise habits. Are there areas where you've become less consistent?

- **Change Your Routine:** Mix up your workout routine or try new activities to challenge your body in different ways.

- **Set Non-Scale Goals:** Focus on non-scale victories like increased energy, improved fitness, or better sleep quality. These can keep you motivated during plateaus.

9. Lack of Support

Challenge: Sometimes, you may not have a supportive network or people who understand your weight loss goals.

Solution:

- **Online Communities:** Join online forums or social media groups dedicated to weight loss and vegetarianism. You can find like-minded individuals who can offer support and advice.

- **Educate Others:** Share information about the benefits of a vegetarian diet and how it aligns with your weight loss goals. Education can help people better understand your choices.

- **Seek Professional Help:** If you're struggling to find support, consider working with a registered dietitian or a therapist who specializes in weight management.

10. Setbacks and Self-Compassion

Challenge: Weight loss journeys are rarely linear, and setbacks are normal.

Solution:

- **Practice Self-Compassion:** Be kind to yourself when you experience setbacks. Avoid self-criticism, and instead, focus on what you can learn from the experience.
- **Learn from Setbacks:** Analyze what led to the setback and use it as an opportunity to adjust your strategies and develop resilience.

- **Stay Persistent:** Understand that setbacks are a part of any journey, but they don't define your overall progress. Keep moving forward with determination.

11. Sustainability

Challenge: Maintaining the changes you've made for the long term can be challenging.

Solution:

- **Lifestyle Approach:** Instead of viewing weight loss as a temporary goal, adopt a lifestyle approach.

Make sustainable changes that you can maintain for the rest of your life.

- **Periodic Reevaluation:** Periodically assess your goals and habits to ensure they align with your long-term health and weight maintenance.

- **Celebrate Successes:** Celebrate your achievements and recognize the positive impact your changes have had on your health and well-being.

In this chapter, we've addressed various challenges that you may encounter during your vegetarian weight loss journey and provided practical solutions to overcome them. Remember that each person's journey is unique, and it's normal to face obstacles along the way. The key is to stay adaptable, patient, and committed to your health and well-being. With the right strategies and mindset, you can achieve your weight loss goals on a vegetarian diet and enjoy a healthier, happier life.

CHAPTER 8

Maintaining Your Vegetarian Weight Loss

Welcome to Chapter 8 of "Vegetarian Weight Loss Success." Congratulations on your journey so far! You've worked hard to achieve your weight loss goals on a vegetarian diet. Now, it's time to discuss how to maintain your progress and embrace a sustainable, healthy lifestyle for the long term. Weight maintenance is a crucial phase of your journey, and this chapter will guide you through it.

1. Embrace a Sustainable Lifestyle

Maintaining your weight loss isn't about returning to old habits; it's about embracing a new, healthier lifestyle. Here's how to do it:

- **Consistency:** Continue practicing the healthy habits you've developed during your weight loss journey, such as balanced eating and regular exercise.
- **Flexibility:** Be open to adapting your routines as

life changes. Flexibility allows you to navigate different situations without derailing your progress.

- **Mindful Choices:** Keep making conscious food choices. Remember that every meal is an opportunity to nourish your body.

2. Set Realistic Goals

Maintaining your weight loss isn't about reaching a specific number on the scale; it's about staying within a healthy range. Setting realistic goals can help you stay motivated:

- **Maintenance Range:** Identify a weight range within which you're comfortable and healthy. This range allows for some natural fluctuations without causing concern.

- **Non-Scale Goals:** Focus on non-scale victories like improved fitness, increased energy, or better sleep quality. These goals can be just as motivating as a number on the scale.

3. Monitor Your Progress

Regularly tracking your progress can help you stay accountable and make necessary adjustments:

- **Weigh-In Routine:** Weigh yourself regularly, but avoid becoming obsessed with daily fluctuations. Weekly or bi-weekly weigh-ins can provide a more accurate picture.

- **Measurements:** Continue tracking body measurements, as changes in inches can be just as important as changes in weight.

- **Keep a Food Journal:** Consider keeping a food journal to stay mindful of your eating habits. It can help you identify areas that need attention.

4. Stay Active

Physical activity remains essential for weight maintenance and overall health:

- **Consistency:** Maintain your exercise routine. Regular activity helps you burn calories and supports a healthy metabolism.

- **Variety:** Keep your workouts interesting by trying new activities or classes. This prevents boredom and helps you stay engaged.

- **Functional Fitness:** Focus on functional fitness to improve your strength and mobility, making daily activities easier and more enjoyable.

5. Balanced Nutrition

Continue to prioritize balanced nutrition to support your health and weight maintenance:

- **Portion Control:** Pay attention to portion sizes, especially when dining out or enjoying treats.

- **Healthy Eating Habits:** Practice mindful eating, listening to your body's hunger and fullness cues. Avoid eating out of boredom or stress.

- **Whole Foods:** Emphasize whole, unprocessed foods in your diet. These provide essential nutrients and promote satiety.

6. Meal Planning and Preparation

Maintain your meal planning and preparation habits, as they're essential for consistency:

- **Batch Cooking:** Continue batch cooking to have healthy meals readily available during busy days.
- **Healthy Snacks:** Keep healthy snacks on hand to avoid impulsive, less nutritious choices.
- **Variety:** Continue experimenting with new recipes and ingredients to keep your meals exciting.

7. Social Support

Lean on your support system for encouragement and accountability:

- **Share Your Goals:** Continue sharing your goals and progress with friends and family who support your journey.

- **Accountability Partners:** Consider having an accountability partner or joining a maintenance-focused group to stay motivated.

8. Manage Stress

Stress can impact your weight and overall well-being. Here's how to manage it:

- **Stress-Reduction Techniques:** Continue using stress-reduction techniques like deep breathing, meditation, or yoga.
- **Prioritize Self-Care:** Make self-care a regular part of your routine to help manage stress and maintain emotional balance.

9. Celebrate Your Success

Take time to celebrate your achievements, both big and small:

- **Acknowledge Milestones:** Recognize the progress you've made and celebrate your successes along the way.
- **Positive Reinforcement:** Use positive self-talk and rewards to reinforce your commitment to a healthy lifestyle.

10. Learn from Setbacks

Setbacks are a natural part of any long-term journey. Here's how to handle them:

- **Resilience:** Develop resilience by viewing setbacks as opportunities for learning and growth.
- **Analysis:** Analyze what led to the setback and adjust your strategies accordingly.
- **Avoid Guilt:** Avoid guilt and self-criticism. Remember that everyone faces challenges on their journey.

11. Seek Professional Guidance

If you find it challenging to maintain your weight loss or have specific concerns about your health, consider seeking professional guidance:

- **Dietitian or Nutritionist:** A registered dietitian can help you create a maintenance plan that suits your unique needs and preferences.

- **Trainer or Coach:** Consider working with a fitness trainer or coach to fine-tune your exercise routine.

- **Medical Evaluation:** If you're experiencing health issues related to weight or nutrition, consult with a healthcare professional for personalized guidance.

12. Stay Informed

Continue educating yourself about nutrition and health to make informed choices:

- **Stay Updated:** Stay informed about the latest research and recommendations regarding vegetarian nutrition and weight management.
- **Expand Your Knowledge:** Consider taking cooking classes, reading books, or attending

seminars related to healthy living.

13. Be Patient and Kind to Yourself

Above all, practice patience and self-compassion:

- **Lifelong Journey:** Understand that weight maintenance is a lifelong journey. There will be ups and downs, but each day is a chance to make healthy choices.

- **Self-Compassion:** Be kind to yourself, especially during challenging moments. Avoid self-criticism and instead focus on your progress and resilience.

- **Celebrate the Journey:** Embrace the journey itself, not just the destination. Enjoy the process of maintaining your health and well-being.

14. Prepare for Life Changes

Life is full of changes, and they can impact your health and weight. Here's how to prepare:

- **Stay Adaptable:** Be flexible and open to adapting

your routines as life circumstances change.

- **Planning Ahead:** Anticipate major life events and plan how you'll continue prioritizing your health through those transitions.

- **Seek Support:** If you're facing significant life changes, consider seeking guidance from a professional or support group.

15. Reflect on Your Journey

Finally, take time to reflect on your journey:

- **Gratitude:** Express gratitude for the progress you've made and the positive changes in your life.

- **Future Goals:** Set new goals or challenges for yourself to keep your journey exciting and motivating.

Remember that maintaining your weight loss is a significant achievement, and it's worth the effort. By embracing a sustainable, healthy lifestyle and staying committed to your well-being, you can enjoy the long-term benefits of your vegetarian weight loss journey. Congratulations on your success!

CHAPTER 9

Navigating Life Transitions and Special Circumstances on a Vegetarian Diet

Life is full of transitions and special circumstances that can present unique challenges when it comes to maintaining a vegetarian diet and a healthy lifestyle. In Chapter 9 of "Vegetarian Weight Loss Success," we'll explore how to navigate these situations while staying true to your dietary preferences and wellness goals.

Whether you're facing changes in your life, dealing with social situations, or managing health considerations, this chapter provides practical guidance for maintaining your vegetarian weight loss success.

1.   Transitioning to Parenthood

Challenge: Becoming a parent is a life-altering transition that can impact your time, energy, and dietary choices.

Solution:

- **Meal Planning:** Prioritize meal planning and

preparation to ensure you have healthy options readily available for yourself and your family.

- **Family-Friendly Recipes:** Explore family-friendly vegetarian recipes that appeal to both adults and children. Involve your kids in meal planning and cooking to encourage healthy eating habits.

- **Seek Support:** Connect with other vegetarian parents for recipe ideas and tips on raising vegetarian children.

2. Traveling as a Vegetarian

Challenge: Traveling, especially to areas with limited vegetarian options, can pose challenges for maintaining your dietary choices.

Solution:

- **Research and Planning:** Before traveling, research vegetarian-friendly restaurants and markets in the area you'll be visiting. Plan your meals in advance whenever possible.
- **Pack Snacks:** Bring healthy vegetarian snacks like nuts, dried fruits, and

granola bars to tide you over
between meals.

- **Learn Local Dishes:**
Embrace the opportunity to
try local vegetarian dishes.
Many cultures have delicious
vegetarian options to
explore.

3. Coping with Stress and Emotional Eating

Challenge: Life stressors can
lead to emotional eating, making it
challenging to maintain a healthy
diet.

Solution:

- **Stress Management:** Practice stress-reduction techniques such as meditation, yoga, or deep breathing exercises to manage emotional eating triggers.

- **Mindful Eating:** When you feel stressed or emotional, take a moment to check in with your body's hunger cues. Are you truly hungry, or are you seeking comfort through food?

- **Seek Support:** Consider speaking with a therapist or counselor to address the underlying emotional factors contributing to emotional eating.

4. Managing Vegetarianism in Social Situations

Challenge: Social situations often revolve around food, and explaining your dietary choices to others can be challenging.

Solution:

- **Effective Communication:** Develop a brief, respectful explanation of your vegetarian lifestyle that you can share when necessary. Emphasize that it's a personal choice for your health and well-being.

- **Offer to Contribute:** When attending gatherings, offer to bring a vegetarian dish to share. This ensures you have something substantial to eat and introduces others to delicious meatless options.

- **Educate and Share:** Share information about the benefits of a vegetarian diet when appropriate, but avoid lecturing or making others uncomfortable.

5. Coping with Special Diets for Medical Reasons

Challenge: Some individuals may need to follow special diets for medical reasons while maintaining a vegetarian lifestyle.

Solution:

- **Consult a Healthcare Professional:** If you have specific medical dietary requirements, consult with a healthcare professional or registered dietitian who can help you navigate your dietary choices.

- **Balance and Adapt:** Work with a healthcare provider to develop a dietary plan that meets both your medical needs and your vegetarian preferences.

- **Educate Yourself:** Educate yourself about vegetarian sources of essential nutrients that are relevant to your medical condition. Stay informed about the foods that are beneficial and those to avoid.

6. Vegetarianism in Athletic Endeavors

Challenge: Maintaining a vegetarian diet while pursuing athletic endeavors can require careful planning to ensure optimal performance and recovery.

Solution:

- **Nutrient Timing:** Pay attention to nutrient timing, ensuring you consume an appropriate balance of carbohydrates, protein, and healthy fats before and after workouts.

- **Protein Needs:** If you're physically active, you may need more protein. Ensure you're getting enough plant-based protein sources to support muscle recovery and growth.

- **Hydration:** Stay well-hydrated, especially during intense physical activity. Water, herbal teas, and sports drinks can help you stay hydrated.

7. Managing a Vegetarian Diet as You Age

Challenge: As you age, your nutritional needs may change, and it can become more challenging to maintain a balanced diet.

Solution:

- **Regular Check-Ups:** Schedule regular check-ups with a healthcare provider who can assess your nutritional status and provide guidance on any necessary dietary adjustments.

- **Fortified Foods:** Consider including fortified foods in your diet to ensure you're getting essential nutrients like vitamin B12 and vitamin D.

- **Balance and Variety:** Continue to prioritize a balanced diet with a variety of fruits, vegetables, whole grains, and plant-based proteins.

8. Coping with Cravings and Temptations

Challenge: Even as an experienced vegetarian, you may still experience cravings for non-vegetarian foods.

Solution:

- **Healthy Substitutes:** Seek out or create vegetarian versions of your favorite non-vegetarian dishes. Today, there are plant-based alternatives for many animal-based products.

- **Mindful Indulgence:** Occasionally indulging in your favorite non-vegetarian foods is okay. Practice moderation and savor these treats when you choose to enjoy them.

- **Stay Hydrated:** Sometimes, thirst can be mistaken for hunger. Drink water when you have a craving to see if it subsides.

9. Navigating Menopause on a Vegetarian Diet

Challenge: Menopause brings hormonal changes that can affect your metabolism and weight.

Maintaining a healthy weight during this transition can be challenging.

Solution:

- **Balanced Diet:** Prioritize a balanced diet with nutrient-dense foods to support your metabolism and overall health.

- **Regular Exercise:** Engage in regular physical activity to help manage weight and reduce symptoms associated with menopause.

- **Consult a Healthcare Provider:** Speak with a healthcare provider or registered dietitian who specializes in women's health to address specific concerns related to menopause and your vegetarian diet.

10. Managing Vegetarianism During Pregnancy and Breastfeeding

Challenge: Pregnancy and breastfeeding require additional nutrients, and it's essential to ensure you and your baby receive proper nutrition while maintaining a vegetarian diet.

Solution:

- **Prenatal Care:** Seek prenatal care early in your pregnancy and discuss your vegetarian diet with a healthcare provider who can recommend appropriate supplements.

- **Balanced Diet:** Pay extra attention to a balanced diet during pregnancy and breastfeeding. Ensure you're getting enough protein, iron, calcium, folic acid, and other essential nutrients.

- **Consult a Dietitian:** Work with a registered dietitian who specializes in prenatal and postnatal nutrition for personalized guidance.

11. Navigating the Vegetarian Diet in Retirement

Challenge: Retirement often brings changes in daily routines and lifestyle, which can impact dietary choices.

Solution:

- **Routine Maintenance:** Maintain healthy eating habits established during your working years. Continue to prioritize a balanced diet and regular physical activity.

- **Social Connections:** Stay connected with friends and family who share your dietary preferences. This can provide social support and help you stay motivated.

- **Regular Check-Ups:** As you age, regular check-ups become even more critical to monitor your health and nutrition.

12. Handling Food Allergies and Sensitivities

Challenge: Food allergies and sensitivities can make it challenging to maintain a vegetarian diet while avoiding specific allergens.

Solution:

- **Identify Safe Alternatives:** Identify safe vegetarian alternatives for foods you're allergic or sensitive to. For example, if you're allergic to soy, explore other plant-based protein sources like beans or lentils.

- **Read Labels:** Always read food labels carefully to avoid potential allergens or irritants. Familiarize yourself with ingredient names that might indicate the presence of allergens.

- **Consult an Allergist:** Work with an allergist to accurately identify and manage your food allergies or sensitivities.

13. Preparing for End-of-Life Dietary Preferences

Challenge: As you approach the end of life, it's essential to communicate your dietary preferences and values to your loved ones and healthcare providers.

Solution:

- **Advance Directives:** Consider creating advance directives or including dietary preferences in your end-of-life plans to ensure your wishes are respected.

- **Open Communication:** Have open and compassionate conversations with your family and healthcare team about your dietary choices and how they align with your values and beliefs.

- **Seek Support:** If you have specific cultural or religious dietary preferences, consult with spiritual leaders or counselors for guidance.

14. Navigating Dietary Changes for Environmental or Ethical Reasons

Challenge: You may decide to adjust your vegetarian diet for environmental or ethical reasons, such as reducing your carbon footprint or supporting sustainable food systems.

Solution:

- **Informed Choices:** Research and make informed choices about the environmental and ethical aspects of your dietary preferences. Explore plant-based foods with lower environmental impacts.

- **Balanced Approach:** Maintain a balanced diet while aligning with your ethical and environmental values. Consult resources and organizations dedicated to sustainable and ethical eating.

- **Advocacy and Engagement:** Consider getting involved in local or global initiatives that promote sustainable and ethical food practices.

15. Reflecting on Your Journey

Challenge: Over time, it's valuable to reflect on your vegetarian weight loss journey and the impact it has had on your life.

Solution:

- **Gratitude:** Express gratitude for the positive changes in your health, well-being, and the environment that your dietary choices have supported.
- **Share Your Story:** Consider sharing your journey with others to

inspire and educate them about the benefits of a vegetarian lifestyle.

- **Future Goals:** Set new goals or challenges for yourself related to your diet and wellness journey.

Navigating life transitions and special circumstances on a vegetarian diet requires adaptability, planning, and a commitment to your health and values. By staying informed, seeking support when needed, and staying true to your dietary preferences, you can continue to enjoy the many benefits of a vegetarian lifestyle throughout all stages of life and diverse circumstances. Remember that your journey is unique, and it's okay to seek guidance from professionals or peers as you navigate these challenges.

CHAPTER 10

Sustaining Your Vegetarian Weight Loss Success for Life

Welcome to the final chapter of "Vegetarian Weight Loss Success." By reaching this point, you've demonstrated dedication, perseverance, and commitment to your health. In Chapter 10, we'll explore the essential principles and strategies for sustaining your vegetarian weight loss success for life. This chapter is about making your achievements permanent, enjoying long-term health benefits, and ensuring that your journey remains fulfilling and sustainable.

1. Embrace the Journey as a Lifestyle

At this stage, it's crucial to acknowledge that your weight loss journey isn't merely a short-term endeavor. It's a lifelong commitment to a healthier, more fulfilling lifestyle. Rather than viewing weight loss as a goal you've achieved, think of it as a path you've chosen to continue walking. Embracing this mindset shift is key to sustaining your success.

- **Consistency:** Continue practicing the habits that have contributed to your success, from mindful eating to regular exercise.
- **Adaptability:** Stay open to adapting your routines and strategies as life circumstances change. Flexibility is essential for long-term success.
- **Enjoyment:** Choose activities, foods, and routines that you genuinely enjoy. Sustainability is easier

when you find pleasure in your choices.

2. Set Realistic and Sustainable Goals

While you may have reached your initial weight loss goals, setting new, realistic, and sustainable objectives is essential for long-term success. These goals can help you stay motivated and focused on your health journey.

- **Maintenance Range:** Establish a weight range within which you're comfortable and healthy. This allows for natural fluctuations without causing concern.

- **Non-Scale Goals:** Shift your focus from the number on the scale to non-scale victories like improved fitness, increased energy, and better sleep quality.

3. Monitor and Adjust Your Progress

Consistently monitoring your progress and making necessary adjustments is an ongoing process. Regular check-ins can help you stay accountable and fine-tune your approach.

- **Regular Weigh-Ins:** Continue to weigh yourself periodically, but avoid becoming obsessed with daily fluctuations.

- **Measurements:** Keep tracking body measurements, as changes in inches can be just as important as changes in weight.

- **Food Journaling:** Consider maintaining a food journal to stay mindful of your eating habits and identify areas that need attention.

4. Maintain an Active Lifestyle

Physical activity remains a cornerstone of long-term weight maintenance and overall well-being. Here's how to keep it an integral part of your life:

- **Consistency:** Maintain your exercise routine. Regular activity helps you burn calories, maintain muscle mass, and support a healthy metabolism.

- **Variety:** Keep your workouts interesting by trying new activities, classes, or outdoor adventures.

Variety prevents boredom and keeps you engaged.

- **Functional Fitness:** Focus on functional fitness exercises that improve your strength, mobility, and balance, enhancing your overall quality of life.

5. Prioritize Balanced Nutrition

Balanced nutrition continues to be vital for sustaining your weight loss success. Consistently making healthy food choices ensures you continue to nourish your body effectively.

- **Portion Control:** Stay mindful of portion sizes, especially when dining out or indulging in treats.

- **Healthy Eating Habits:** Continue practicing mindful eating by listening to your body's hunger and fullness cues. Avoid emotional or stress-driven eating.

- **Whole Foods:** Emphasize whole, unprocessed foods in your diet. These provide essential nutrients and promote satiety.

6. Plan and Prepare Your Meals

Maintaining your meal planning and preparation habits ensures you have healthy options readily available during busy days.

- **Batch Cooking:** Keep batch cooking as part of your routine. Preparing large quantities of staple foods and freezing portions can save time and money.

- **Healthy Snacks:** Maintain the habit of having healthy snacks on hand to prevent impulsive, less nutritious choices.

- **Variety:** Continue experimenting with new

recipes and ingredients to keep your meals exciting and satisfying.

7. Cultivate a Supportive Network

Lean on your support system to stay motivated and accountable as you continue your journey.

- **Share Your Goals:** Keep sharing your goals and progress with friends and family who support your health journey.
- **Accountability Partners:** Consider having an accountability partner or

joining a maintenance-focused group. These connections can provide encouragement and motivation.

8. Manage Stress Effectively

Stress can impact your weight and overall well-being. Continue to prioritize effective stress management techniques:

- **Stress-Reduction Techniques:** Maintain practices like meditation, yoga, or deep breathing exercises to manage stress effectively.

- **Prioritize Self-Care:** Regularly include self-care activities in your routine, such as relaxation, hobbies, or spending time in nature.

9. Celebrate Your Successes

Don't forget to celebrate your achievements, no matter how big or small. Positive reinforcement can help you maintain motivation and dedication.

- **Acknowledge Milestones:** Recognize the progress you've made and celebrate your successes along the way.

- **Reward Yourself:** Use positive self-talk and rewards to reinforce your commitment to a healthy lifestyle.

10. Learn from Setbacks

Setbacks are a natural part of any long-term journey. How you respond to them is crucial to sustaining your success.

- **Develop Resilience:** View setbacks as opportunities for learning and growth. Developing resilience will help you bounce back from challenges.

- **Analyze and Adjust:** When setbacks occur, analyze what led to them and adjust your strategies accordingly.

- **Avoid Guilt:** Refrain from self-criticism or guilt. Remember that everyone faces obstacles on their path to health.

11. Seek Professional Guidance When Needed

If you find it challenging to sustain your weight loss or have specific concerns about your health, consider seeking professional guidance:

- **Dietitian or Nutritionist:** A registered dietitian can help you create a maintenance plan tailored to your unique needs and preferences.

- **Trainer or Coach:** Working with a fitness trainer or coach can help you fine-tune your exercise routine and stay motivated.

- **Medical Evaluation:** If you experience health issues related to weight or nutrition, consult with a healthcare professional for personalized guidance.

12. Stay Informed and Educated

Continue educating yourself about nutrition, health, and wellness to make informed choices:

- **Stay Updated:** Stay informed about the latest research and recommendations regarding vegetarian nutrition, weight management, and overall health.

- **Expand Your Knowledge:** Consider taking cooking classes, reading books, or attending seminars related to healthy living.

13. Be Patient and Kind to Yourself

Above all, practice patience and self-compassion:

- **Long-Term Perspective:** Understand that weight maintenance is a lifelong journey. There will be ups and downs, but each day offers a chance to make healthy choices.
- **Self-Compassion:** Be kind to yourself, especially during challenging moments. Avoid

self-criticism and instead focus on your progress and resilience.

- **Celebrate the Journey:** Embrace the journey itself, not just the destination. Continue to enjoy the process of maintaining your health and well-being.

14. Prepare for Life Changes

Life is full of changes, and they can impact your health and weight. Here's how to prepare:

- **Stay Adaptable:** Be flexible and open to adapting

your routines as life circumstances change.

- **Planning Ahead:** Anticipate major life events and plan how you'll continue prioritizing your health through those transitions.

- **Seek Support:** If you're facing significant life changes, consider seeking guidance from a professional or support group.

15. Reflect on Your Journey

Take time to reflect on your incredible journey:

- **Gratitude:** Express gratitude for the progress you've made and the positive changes in your life, health, and well-being.

- **Share Your Story:** Consider sharing your journey with others to inspire and educate them about the benefits of a vegetarian lifestyle.

- **Future Goals:** Set new goals or challenges for yourself to keep your journey exciting and motivating.

In this concluding chapter, we've explored the essential principles and strategies for sustaining your vegetarian weight loss success for life. Remember that your journey is a dynamic and ongoing process, and your commitment to your health is a lifelong endeavor. Embrace the lifestyle, set realistic goals, stay consistent, and be kind to yourself as you continue to enjoy the lasting benefits of your vegetarian weight loss journey. Congratulations on your incredible achievement!

CONCLUSION

In concluding "Vegetarian Weight Loss Success," it's essential to celebrate the remarkable journey you've undertaken. Throughout this book, we've explored the principles, strategies, and wisdom needed to embark on a transformative path towards better health and well-being through a vegetarian diet. Your dedication and commitment to this journey are commendable, and the benefits you've gained are both inspiring and life-changing.

As you close this chapter of your reading, remember that this book isn't just a manual for weight loss. It's a testament to the power of choice, the strength of determination, and the resilience of the human spirit. It's a reminder that positive change is possible, and that you have the capacity to take control of your health and happiness.

Your journey doesn't end here. In fact, it's just beginning. Your commitment to a vegetarian lifestyle, along with the knowledge and tools you've gained, will serve you well as you continue to navigate the complex landscape of health and nutrition. The principles discussed in this book aren't just for losing weight; they're for living a vibrant, balanced, and fulfilling life.

As you move forward, remember these key takeaways:

1. **Lifestyle, Not Diet:** Embrace your vegetarian lifestyle as a long-term commitment to your health and the well-being of the planet. It's not just a diet; it's a way of life.

2. **Realistic Goals:** Set achievable and sustainable

goals for yourself. Weight loss is just one facet of your journey; overall health and well-being are the ultimate rewards.

3. **Mindful Choices:** Practice mindfulness in your eating habits and daily life. Listen to your body's cues, and make choices that nourish both your body and your soul.

4. **Stay Active:** Physical activity is a pillar of your health. Keep moving, exploring, and challenging yourself physically, not just

to lose weight but to live a more vibrant life.

5. **Balanced Nutrition:** Prioritize balanced nutrition by choosing whole, unprocessed foods and practicing portion control. Food is your fuel; make it count.

6. **Planning and Preparation:** Meal planning and preparation are your allies in maintaining a healthy lifestyle. They save you time, money, and keep you on track.

7. **Support System:** Lean on your support system. Share your journey with loved ones who encourage and uplift you. You're not alone on this path.

8. **Resilience:** Understand that setbacks are a natural part of any journey. Your ability to bounce back and adapt is a testament to your strength.

9. **Continuous Learning:** Keep educating yourself about nutrition, health, and wellness. Knowledge is your power, and it evolves over time.

10.   **Self-Compassion:**
Finally, be kind to yourself. This journey is as much about self-love as it is about health. Celebrate your successes, and don't dwell on occasional missteps.

In closing, remember that your journey is unique, and your story is still being written. "Vegetarian Weight Loss Success" is not the end; it's a guide to a lifelong adventure in health and well-being. As you turn the final page, embrace the possibilities that lie ahead with enthusiasm, knowing that your path is one of vitality, compassion, and lasting success.

Congratulations on your incredible achievements, and may your journey be filled with continued health, happiness, and fulfillment.